BREAST CANCER SURVIVAL GUIDE

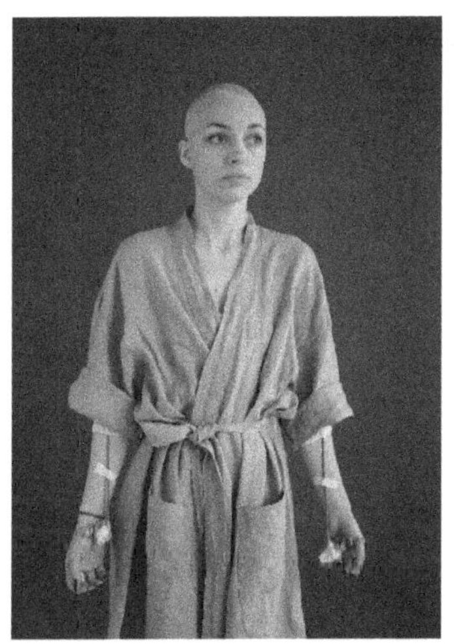

A full detailed Guide on Breast Cancer diagnosis, treatment, and absolute recovery.

By

Bradley P. Taylor

ABOUT THE BOOK

"Breast Cancer Survival Guide" is a beacon of hope and practical wisdom for anyone grappling with the complexities of a breast cancer diagnosis. Authored by experts in oncology and enriched with firsthand accounts from survivors, this guidebook offers a roadmap through every stage of the journey, from initial diagnosis to survivorship.

At its core, the book provides clear explanations of medical terminologies, treatment options, and potential side effects, empowering readers to make informed decisions about their health. It covers the latest advancements in breast cancer research and therapies, ensuring that the information is up-to-date and reliable.

Beyond medical advice, the guide delves into the emotional and psychological aspects of coping with breast cancer. It offers strategies for managing stress, maintaining a positive outlook, and seeking support from friends, family, and support groups. Practical tips on nutrition, exercise, and self-care are also included to help optimize overall well-being during treatment and recovery.

Throughout its pages, "Breast Cancer Survival Guide" emphasizes resilience and empowerment. It celebrates the strength of survivors and provides encouragement to those navigating the uncertainties of diagnosis and treatment. By combining medical expertise with compassionate guidance, this book serves as a companion for individuals facing breast cancer, equipping them with the knowledge and resources needed to navigate their journey with courage and hope.

TABLE OF CONTENT

CONCLUSION

Introduction

1.1 Definition of Breast Cancer

Breast cancer is a disease in which malignant (cancer) cells form in the tissues of the breast. This process typically begins in the cells of the ducts (tubes that carry milk from the lobules to the nipple) or the lobules (glands that produce milk). In some cases, cancer may also start in the stromal tissues, which include the fatty and fibrous connective tissues of the breast. The development of breast cancer involves a complex interplay of genetic, environmental, and lifestyle factors.

There are several types of breast cancer, each defined by the specific cells in the breast that become cancerous. The most common types are ductal carcinoma in situ (DCIS), which is a non-invasive cancer where cells inside the ducts have changed to cancer cells but have not spread to surrounding breast tissue, and invasive ductal carcinoma (IDC), which begins in the milk ducts and invades nearby tissues. Another type is invasive lobular carcinoma (ILC), which starts in the lobules and spreads to nearby tissues.

Breast cancer can be classified based on hormone receptor status and the presence of certain proteins. Hormone receptor-positive cancers have cells that contain receptors for the hormones estrogen and/or progesterone, which can promote cancer growth. HER2-positive breast cancers have an excess of the human epidermal growth factor receptor 2 protein, which also stimulates cancer growth. Triple-negative breast cancer lacks receptors for estrogen, progesterone, and HER2, and is often more aggressive and harder to treat.

Risk factors for breast cancer include gender (it is far more common in women than in men), age (the risk increases as one gets older), genetic mutations (such as BRCA1 and BRCA2), family history of breast cancer, personal history of breast cancer or certain non-cancerous breast diseases, dense breast tissue, radiation exposure, and certain lifestyle factors like alcohol consumption, obesity, and lack of physical activity.

Diagnosis of breast cancer typically involves imaging tests such as mammograms, ultrasounds, and MRIs, followed by a biopsy to examine tissue samples under a microscope. Treatment options vary depending on the stage and type of breast cancer and may include surgery, radiation therapy, chemotherapy, hormone therapy, and targeted therapy.

Early detection and advances in treatment have significantly improved the prognosis for many individuals with breast cancer, making it possible to manage the disease effectively and improve survival rates. Regular screenings and awareness of breast cancer signs and symptoms are crucial in catching the disease early and improving outcomes.

1.2 Risk Factors For Breast Cancer

Breast cancer is influenced by a variety of risk factors, encompassing genetic, environmental, and lifestyle elements. Understanding these factors can aid in identifying individuals at higher risk and implementing preventive measures.

1. Genetic Factors: One of the most significant risk factors for breast cancer is genetics. Mutations in specific genes, particularly BRCA1 and BRCA2, substantially increase the risk. Women with these mutations have a 45-65% chance of developing breast cancer by age 70.

Additionally, a family history of breast cancer, especially in first-degree relatives (mother, sister, daughter), increases risk. Genetic testing and counseling are recommended for those with a strong family history.

2. Hormonal and Reproductive Factors: Hormonal influences play a crucial role. Early menarche (before age 12) and late menopause (after age 55) prolong exposure to estrogen and increase risk. Nulliparity (never having given birth) or having the first child after age 30 also heighten risk. Prolonged use of hormone replacement therapy (HRT) during menopause, especially combined estrogen-progesterone therapy, is linked to higher breast cancer incidence.

3. Age and Gender: Age is a primary risk factor, with most breast cancers occurring in women over 50. Although men can develop breast cancer, it is about 100 times more common in women. Female gender remains the most significant risk factor for the disease.

4. Personal History: A personal history of breast cancer increases the likelihood of developing new cancer in the other breast or another part of the same breast. Certain non-cancerous breast conditions, such as atypical hyperplasia or lobular carcinoma in situ (LCIS), also elevate risk.

5. Lifestyle Factors: Several lifestyle factors influence breast cancer risk. Obesity, particularly postmenopausal, raises risk due to increased estrogen production from fat tissue. Alcohol consumption is another significant factor; even moderate drinking can increase risk. Physical inactivity is associated with higher risk, whereas regular exercise is protective.

6. Radiation Exposure: Exposure to radiation, particularly to the chest area during childhood or young adulthood (such as treatment for Hodgkin's lymphoma), increases breast cancer risk. The risk is higher if the radiation exposure occurred during periods of rapid breast development.

7. Environmental Factors: While the exact impact of environmental factors is still being studied, exposure to certain chemicals and pollutants, including those that mimic estrogen, may increase breast cancer risk. Lifestyle and environmental modifications, alongside regular screenings, can help mitigate some of these risks.

8. Breast Density: Women with dense breast tissue have a higher risk of breast cancer. Dense tissue can also make it harder to detect cancer on mammograms, complicating early diagnosis.

9. Socioeconomic Factors: Socioeconomic status can indirectly influence breast cancer risk through access to healthcare, screening, and awareness. Women with higher socioeconomic status are more likely to have better access to preventive care and early detection services.

1.3 Types and Stages of Breast Cancer.

Breast cancer encompasses various types, each with distinct characteristics, origins, and treatment approaches. Understanding these types is crucial for accurate diagnosis and effective management.

1.3.1 Types of Breast Cancer

1. Ductal Carcinoma In Situ (DCIS): DCIS is a non-invasive breast cancer confined to the milk ducts. It is considered the earliest form of breast cancer, as the cancer cells have not spread beyond the ducts into surrounding breast tissue. While not life-threatening, DCIS can increase the risk of developing invasive breast cancer. Treatment typically involves surgery (lumpectomy or mastectomy) and sometimes radiation therapy to reduce recurrence risk.

2. Invasive Ductal Carcinoma (IDC): IDC is the most common type of breast cancer, accounting

for about 80% of cases. It begins in the milk ducts and invades the surrounding breast tissue. IDC can metastasize to other parts of the body through the lymphatic system and bloodstream. Treatment options include surgery, radiation therapy, chemotherapy, hormone therapy, and targeted therapy, depending on the stage and characteristics of the tumor.

3. Invasive Lobular Carcinoma (ILC): ILC starts in the lobules (milk-producing glands) and spreads to surrounding tissues. It accounts for about 10-15% of invasive breast cancers. ILC can be more challenging to detect through mammograms due to its tendency to grow in a line rather than forming a lump. Treatment is similar to IDC and may include surgery, radiation therapy, chemotherapy, hormone therapy, and targeted therapy.

4. Triple-Negative Breast Cancer (TNBC): TNBC lacks estrogen receptors (ER), progesterone receptors (PR), and HER2 protein. It is more aggressive and harder to treat since

hormone therapy and HER2-targeted treatments are ineffective. TNBC is more common in younger women and those with BRCA1 gene mutations. Treatment often involves a combination of surgery, chemotherapy, and radiation therapy.

5. HER2-Positive Breast Cancer: This type of breast cancer tests positive for the human epidermal growth factor receptor 2 (HER2), which promotes cancer cell growth. HER2-positive cancers tend to grow and spread faster than HER2-negative cancers. However, they often respond well to targeted therapies like trastuzumab (Herceptin) and pertuzumab (Perjeta), in addition to surgery, chemotherapy, and radiation.

6. Hormone Receptor-Positive Breast Cancer: These cancers have cells with receptors for estrogen (ER-positive) and/or progesterone (PR-positive). They grow in response to these hormones. Hormone receptor-positive breast cancers are typically treated with hormone

therapy (such as tamoxifen or aromatase inhibitors) to block the hormones or lower their levels, in addition to other treatments like surgery, radiation, and chemotherapy.

7. Inflammatory Breast Cancer (IBC): IBC is a rare but aggressive type of breast cancer that causes the breast to become red, swollen, and warm due to cancer cells blocking lymph vessels in the skin. It is often mistaken for an infection. Treatment usually involves chemotherapy to shrink the tumor, followed by surgery and radiation therapy.

8. Paget's Disease of the Breast: Paget's disease affects the skin of the nipple and areola and is often associated with underlying DCIS or invasive breast cancer. Symptoms include redness, scaliness, and irritation of the nipple skin. Treatment typically includes surgery (mastectomy or lumpectomy) and may involve radiation therapy.

1.3.2 Stages of Breast Cancer

Breast cancer staging is essential for determining the extent of cancer spread and guiding treatment. The stages range from 0 to IV, based on tumor size, lymph node involvement, and metastasis.

1. Stage 0: Also known as carcinoma in situ, this stage includes ductal carcinoma in situ (DCIS), where cancer cells are confined to the ducts or lobules and have not invaded surrounding tissues.

2. Stage I: An early stage of invasive cancer, with tumors up to 2 cm. Stage IA indicates no lymph node involvement, while stage IB may involve small clusters of cancer cells in nearby lymph nodes.

3. Stage II: Divided into IIA and IIB. Stage IIA involves tumors 2-5 cm or smaller tumors that have spread to 1-3 axillary lymph nodes. Stage

IIB includes larger tumors (2-5 cm) with minor lymph node involvement or tumors larger than 5 cm without lymph node involvement.

4. Stage III: Known as locally advanced cancer, it is subdivided into IIIA, IIIB, and IIIC. This stage involves larger tumors or extensive lymph node involvement, and cancer may have spread to nearby tissues such as the chest wall or skin.

5. Stage IV: Also known as metastatic breast cancer, stage IV indicates cancer has spread to distant organs such as bones, liver, lungs, or brain. Treatment at this stage focuses on controlling the disease and improving quality of life.

Early detection and accurate staging are critical for effective treatment and better outcomes.

CHAPTER 2

Understanding Breast Anatomy And Function

2.1 Overview Of Breast

The human breast is a complex organ primarily composed of glandular, fatty, and connective tissues. While both men and women have breast tissue, it is far more developed in women and serves a critical role in lactation and nurturing offspring. The breast's structure, function, and associated conditions are essential areas of study in medicine, particularly in understanding diseases such as breast cancer.

2.2 Anatomy And Function Of The Breast

Anatomy of the Breast

The breast is located on the chest wall and extends from the collarbone down to the middle of the ribcage. It consists of several key components:

- Lobules: These are small, glandular structures that produce milk. Women typically have 15-20 lobes in each breast, further divided into smaller lobules.

- Ducts: Milk produced in the lobules is carried to the nipple through a network of ducts. These ducts converge at the nipple, which is the outlet for breastfeeding.

- Fatty Tissue: This tissue surrounds the lobules and ducts, providing shape and size to the breast. The amount of fatty tissue varies among individuals, influencing breast size and density.

- Connective Tissue: Ligaments and fibrous connective tissue provide support and structure to the breast, maintaining its shape and position on the chest wall.

- Blood Vessels and Lymphatics: The breast is well-supplied with blood vessels that nourish the tissue. The lymphatic system, consisting of lymph nodes and vessels, plays a crucial role in immune defense and fluid balance.

- Nerves: Sensory nerves in the breast and nipple respond to stimuli, including touch and temperature changes, contributing to both functional and sensory aspects of the breast.

Function of the Breast

The primary biological function of the female breast is to produce and deliver milk to nourish infants, a process known as lactation. During pregnancy, hormonal changes stimulate the growth and development of the mammary glands and ducts. After childbirth, the hormone prolactin promotes milk production, while oxytocin triggers the release of milk during breastfeeding.

2.3 Breast Development

Breast development occurs in several stages:

1. Fetal Development: Basic structures form during fetal growth.
2. Puberty: Estrogen and other hormones trigger the growth of breast tissue, ducts, and lobules, leading to the development of mature breasts.
3. Menstrual Cycle: Hormonal fluctuations during the menstrual cycle cause temporary changes in breast size and tenderness.
4. Pregnancy and Lactation: Significant changes occur to prepare for and sustain milk production.
5. Menopause: Declining hormone levels lead to a reduction in glandular tissue and an increase in fatty tissue.

- **Common Conditions and Diseases**

Understanding breast anatomy and function is essential for recognizing and addressing various conditions that can affect breast health:

1. Breast Cancer: The most significant concern, it arises from the cells of the ducts or lobules. Early detection through regular screening is crucial for effective treatment.
2. Fibrocystic Breast Changes: These benign changes can cause lumps, pain, and tenderness, often related to hormonal fluctuations.
3. Mastitis: An infection of the breast tissue, commonly occurring during breastfeeding, causing pain, redness, and swelling.
4. Gynecomastia: The enlargement of breast tissue in men, usually due to hormonal imbalances.
5. Breast Cysts: Fluid-filled sacs within the breast, often benign but sometimes requiring evaluation to rule out malignancy.

Importance of Breast Health

Maintaining breast health involves regular self-examinations, clinical check-ups, and screenings such as mammograms. Awareness of changes in breast tissue and timely consultation with healthcare providers can aid in early detection and treatment of breast conditions, improving outcomes and overall health.

The breast is a vital organ with complex anatomy and functions essential for reproduction and nurturing. Its health is influenced by a myriad of factors, including hormonal changes, genetic predispositions, and lifestyle choices. Understanding the structure and function of the breast aids in recognizing and managing conditions that affect this critical organ, emphasizing the importance of regular health maintenance and screening.

Chapter 3

Causes and Mechanisms of Breast Cancer.

Breast cancer develops when cells in the breast grow uncontrollably, forming a tumor. This process is driven by genetic mutations and influenced by various risk factors. Understanding the causes and mechanisms behind breast cancer can help in developing prevention strategies and targeted treatments.

3.1 Genetic Mutations

- **Inherited Mutations:**

BRCA1 and BRCA2: These are the most well-known genes associated with an increased risk of breast cancer. Mutations in these genes impair their ability to repair DNA damage, leading to cell growth and cancer development. Women with BRCA1 or BRCA2 mutations have a significantly higher lifetime risk of breast and ovarian cancer.

Other Genetic Mutations: Mutations in genes such as TP53, PTEN, and PALB2 also increase breast cancer risk but are less common than BRCA mutations.

- **Acquired Mutations:**

Most breast cancers are caused by acquired mutations that occur during a person's lifetime rather than inherited. These mutations can be influenced by environmental factors, lifestyle choices, and random errors in DNA replication.

3.2 Hormonal Influence

Hormones, particularly estrogen and progesterone, play a crucial role in breast cancer development. Hormone receptor-positive breast cancers have cells that contain receptors for these hormones, which can promote cancer growth. Factors that increase hormone levels or prolong exposure, such as early menstruation, late menopause, and hormone replacement therapy, can elevate breast cancer risk.

3.3 Environmental and Lifestyle Factors

- Radiation Exposure: Exposure to ionizing radiation, particularly during childhood or young adulthood, increases the risk of developing breast cancer later in life. This is because radiation can cause DNA damage and mutations in breast cells.
- Diet and Physical Activity: A diet high in saturated fats and low in fruits and vegetables, obesity, and lack of physical activity are linked to an increased risk of breast cancer. These factors can influence hormone levels, inflammation, and insulin resistance, contributing to cancer development.
- Alcohol Consumption: Alcohol intake is a known risk factor for breast cancer. It can increase estrogen levels and cause DNA damage, leading to cancerous changes in breast cells.

3.4 Mechanisms of Tumor Development

1. Cell Cycle Dysregulation: Normal cells follow a regulated cycle of growth, division, and death. In cancer cells, mutations disrupt this cycle, leading to uncontrolled growth and division. Key regulators like p53 (a tumor suppressor protein) and cyclin-dependent kinases can be altered, promoting cancer development.

2. DNA Repair Deficiency: Healthy cells have mechanisms to repair DNA damage. Mutations in genes responsible for DNA repair (like BRCA1 and BRCA2) lead to accumulation of genetic errors, contributing to cancer initiation and progression.

3. Angiogenesis: Tumors require a blood supply to grow. They can stimulate the formation of new blood vessels (angiogenesis) to obtain oxygen and nutrients. This process is driven by factors like VEGF (vascular endothelial growth factor).

4. Metastasis: Breast cancer cells can spread from the primary tumor to other parts of the body through the bloodstream or lymphatic system. Metastasis involves multiple steps, including local invasion, intravasation, survival in circulation, extravasation, and colonization of distant organs.

Breast cancer arises from a combination of genetic mutations, hormonal influences, and environmental and lifestyle factors. Understanding these causes and mechanisms is essential for developing effective prevention, early detection, and targeted treatment strategies.

Chapter 4

Signs, Symptoms and Diagnosis of Breast Cancer

4.1 Signs and Symptoms of Breast Cancer

Breast cancer can present with various signs and symptoms, some of which are subtle and easily overlooked. Early detection is crucial for successful treatment and improved outcomes. Understanding the common and less common signs and symptoms of breast cancer can help individuals seek medical attention promptly.

4.1.1 Common Signs and Symptoms

1. Lump or Mass: The most common symptom of breast cancer is a new lump or mass in the breast. These lumps are often painless, hard, and have irregular edges, but they can also be soft, round, or tender. Not all lumps are cancerous, but any new or unusual mass should be evaluated by a healthcare provider.

2. Changes in Breast Shape or Size: Unexplained changes in the size, shape, or appearance of the breast may indicate breast cancer. This can include swelling of all or part of the breast, even if no lump is felt.

3. Skin Changes: Skin dimpling or puckering, often described as resembling the texture of an orange peel (peau d'orange), can be a sign of breast cancer. Redness, scaling, or thickening of the breast skin or nipple can also occur.

4. Nipple Changes: Changes in the nipple, such as inversion (turning inward), discharge (other than breast milk), or pain, can be warning signs. Nipple discharge can be clear, bloody, or another color.

5. Pain: While most breast cancers are not painful in the early stages, some individuals may experience breast pain or discomfort. Persistent pain that does not fluctuate with the menstrual cycle should be evaluated.

4.1.2. Less Common Signs and Symptoms

1. **Swelling or Lump in the Armpit:** Swelling or a lump in the lymph nodes under the arm or around the collarbone can indicate the spread of breast cancer to these areas. This can occur even before the original tumor in the breast is large enough to be felt.

2. **Changes in Breast Texture:** Any noticeable change in the feel of the breast, such as thickening or the presence of unusual texture, should be examined.

3. **Unexplained Weight Loss:** While not specific to breast cancer, unexplained weight loss can sometimes be a sign of advanced cancer.

4. Bone Pain or Fractures: In cases where breast cancer has metastasized, individuals may experience bone pain or fractures, particularly in the back, hips, or ribs.

4.2 Importance of Regular Screening

Regular screening is vital because breast cancer may not cause noticeable symptoms in its early stages. Mammograms, clinical breast exams, and breast self-exams play a critical role in early detection. Women should be aware of how their breasts normally look and feel and report any changes to their healthcare provider immediately.

Recognizing the signs and symptoms of breast cancer is crucial for early diagnosis and treatment. Awareness and regular screening can lead to early detection, significantly improving the chances of successful treatment and survival. If any unusual changes or symptoms are noticed, it is important to seek medical evaluation promptly.

4.3 Diagnosis of Breast Cancer

Diagnosing breast cancer involves a comprehensive approach combining clinical evaluation, imaging techniques, and biopsy procedures. Early and accurate diagnosis is crucial for effective treatment and improving survival rates. Here is an overview of the diagnostic process for breast cancer.

- **Clinical Examination**

The diagnostic process often begins with a clinical breast exam, where a healthcare provider palpates the breasts and surrounding areas, including the undcrarms and collarbone, to check for lumps, abnormalities, or changes in breast tissue. They will also ask about the patient's medical history, symptoms, and any family history of breast cancer.

- **Imaging Techniques**

Imaging plays a pivotal role in detecting and evaluating breast abnormalities. Common imaging techniques include:

1. Mammography: Mammography is the most common screening tool for breast cancer. It uses low-dose X-rays to create detailed images of the breast. Regular mammograms can detect tumors that are too small to be felt and identify microcalcifications that may indicate the presence of cancer.

2. Ultrasound: Breast ultrasound uses sound waves to produce images of the breast tissue. It is often used to further evaluate abnormalities found on a mammogram or physical exam, distinguishing between solid masses and fluid-filled cysts.

3. Magnetic Resonance Imaging (MRI): Breast MRI provides detailed images using magnetic fields and radio waves. It is particularly useful for evaluating the extent of cancer in dense breast tissue, assessing the size of tumors, and checking for additional tumors in the same or opposite breast.

- **Biopsy Procedures**

If imaging studies suggest the presence of cancer, a biopsy is performed to obtain tissue samples for histopathological analysis. There are several types of biopsy procedures:

1. Fine-Needle Aspiration (FNA): A thin needle is used to extract fluid or cells from a suspicious area. FNA is minimally invasive and can determine if a lump is a cyst or a solid mass.

2. Core Needle Biopsy: A larger needle is used to remove a core of tissue from the suspicious area. This method provides more tissue for examination and is more accurate than FNA.

3. Surgical Biopsy: In some cases, a portion (incisional biopsy) or the entire lump (excisional biopsy) is surgically removed for examination. This is more invasive but provides a larger sample for definitive diagnosis.

- **Pathological Analysis**

The tissue obtained from a biopsy is examined under a microscope by a pathologist. The analysis determines whether the cells are cancerous and identifies the type and grade of cancer. Additional tests, such as hormone receptor tests and HER2 status, are conducted to guide treatment decisions.

- **Molecular Testing**

Molecular tests, such as Oncotype DX or MammaPrint, may be performed on the biopsy sample to assess the risk of recurrence and guide treatment choices. These tests analyze the activity of specific genes associated with cancer growth and behavior.

- **Staging**

Once a diagnosis is confirmed, staging is performed to determine the extent of cancer spread. Staging involves a combination of physical exams, imaging tests (such as CT scans, bone scans, and PET scans), and sometimes additional biopsies of lymph nodes or other areas.

The diagnosis of breast cancer involves a combination of clinical evaluation, imaging, biopsy procedures, and pathological analysis. Early detection through regular screening and prompt evaluation of symptoms can significantly improve treatment outcomes and survival rates. If breast cancer is suspected, timely and accurate diagnosis is essential for effective management and care.

CHAPTER 5

Treatment Options for Breast Cancer

Breast cancer treatment is multifaceted, involving a combination of local and systemic therapies tailored to the individual patient's type, stage, and specific characteristics of the cancer. Here is an overview of the main treatment options:

5.1 Surgery

Surgery is often the first line of treatment for breast cancer and aims to remove the tumor from the breast.

- Lumpectomy: Also known as breast-conserving surgery, a lumpectomy involves removing the cancerous lump and a margin of surrounding healthy tissue. This option is typically followed by radiation therapy to eradicate any remaining cancer cells.

- Mastectomy: A mastectomy involves removing the entire breast. There are various types, including total mastectomy (removal of the whole breast) and modified radical mastectomy (removal of the breast and some lymph nodes).

- Sentinel Lymph Node Biopsy: This procedure involves removing a few sentinel lymph nodes (the first nodes to which cancer cells are likely to spread) to check for metastasis. If cancer is found, further lymph nodes may be removed in an axillary lymph node dissection.

5.2 Radiation Therapy

Radiation therapy uses high-energy rays to target and destroy cancer cells. It is commonly used after surgery, especially lumpectomy, to kill any remaining cancer cells in the breast, chest wall, or axilla (underarm area). Types of radiation therapy include:

- External Beam Radiation: This is the most common type, where radiation is delivered from a machine outside the body.

- Brachytherapy: This involves placing radioactive sources inside the breast near the tumor site, often used as a boost in conjunction with external beam radiation.

5.3 Chemotherapy

Chemotherapy involves using drugs to kill cancer cells or stop their growth. It can be administered before surgery (neoadjuvant chemotherapy) to shrink tumors or after surgery (adjuvant chemotherapy) to eliminate any remaining cancer cells. Chemotherapy is particularly effective for aggressive or advanced-stage cancers and typically involves a combination of drugs over several cycles.

5.4 Hormone Therapy

Hormone therapy is used for hormone receptor-positive breast cancers, which grow in response to estrogen or progesterone. Treatments include:

- Selective Estrogen Receptor Modulators (SERMs): Drugs like tamoxifen block estrogen receptors on breast cancer cells, preventing estrogen from promoting cancer growth.

- Aromatase Inhibitors: These drugs, such as anastrozole, letrozole, and exemestane, reduce estrogen production in postmenopausal women.

- Ovarian Suppression: In premenopausal women, treatments like leuprolide or surgery to remove the ovaries can lower estrogen levels.

5.5 Targeted Therapy

Targeted therapy focuses on specific molecules involved in cancer growth. Common targets include HER2, a protein that promotes the growth of cancer cells. Drugs like trastuzumab (Herceptin) and pertuzumab target HER2-positive breast cancers. Other targeted therapies include CDK4/6 inhibitors (palbociclib) and PARP inhibitors (olaparib) for BRCA-mutated cancers.

5.6 Immunotherapy

Immunotherapy enhances the body's immune system to fight cancer. Pembrolizumab, an immune checkpoint inhibitor, has shown promise in treating certain types of breast cancer, especially triple-negative breast cancer.

5.7 Clinical Trials

Clinical trials offer access to cutting-edge treatments and innovative therapies that are not yet widely available. Participation in clinical trials can provide patients with new options and contribute to advancing breast cancer treatment.

The treatment of breast cancer involves a comprehensive approach that combines surgery, radiation therapy, chemotherapy, hormone therapy, targeted therapy, and immunotherapy. The choice of treatment depends on various factors, including the type and stage of cancer, genetic factors, and patient preferences. Advances in personalized medicine continue to improve outcomes and provide hope for those affected by breast cancer.

CHAPTER 6

Managing Treatment Side Effects of Breast Cancer

Breast cancer treatments, while essential for combating the disease, often come with side effects that can impact a patient's quality of life. Managing these side effects effectively is crucial for maintaining overall health and well-being during and after treatment. Here's an overview of common side effects and strategies to manage them:

6.1 Chemotherapy Side Effects

- **Nausea and Vomiting:** Antiemetic medications, dietary adjustments, and small, frequent meals can help control nausea and vomiting. Staying hydrated and avoiding strong odors or spicy foods may also be beneficial.

- **Hair Loss (Alopecia):** Hair loss can be distressing, but using gentle hair care products, wearing wigs, scarves, or hats, and considering scalp cooling caps during treatment can help manage this side effect.
- **Fatigue:** Rest, moderate exercise, and a balanced diet can alleviate fatigue. Prioritizing activities and conserving energy for essential tasks can also be helpful.
- **Infection Risk:** Chemotherapy can lower white blood cell counts, increasing infection risk. Patients should practice good hygiene, avoid crowded places, and promptly report any signs of infection to their healthcare provider.

6.2 Radiation Therapy Side Effects

- **Skin Changes:** Radiation can cause skin irritation, redness, and peeling. Gentle skin care routines, moisturizing, and avoiding tight clothing can help manage these effects. Using prescribed topical treatments can also provide relief.
- **Fatigue**: Similar to chemotherapy, managing fatigue involves rest, balanced nutrition, and light exercise. Stress reduction techniques like yoga and meditation can further alleviate fatigue.
- **Breast Swelling:** Wearing a supportive bra and avoiding heavy lifting can reduce discomfort from breast swelling. Ice packs and over-the-counter pain relief may also be recommended.

6.3 Hormone Therapy Side Effects

- Hot Flashes: Dressing in layers, keeping cool, and avoiding triggers like spicy foods can help manage hot flashes. Medications or supplements may also be prescribed.
- **Bone Health:** Hormone therapies can affect bone density. Ensuring adequate calcium and vitamin D intake, engaging in weight-bearing exercises, and discussing bone density monitoring with a healthcare provider are crucial steps.

6.4 Targeted Therapy Side Effects

- Cardiotoxicity: Some targeted therapies, like those for HER2-positive breast cancer, can affect heart function. Regular monitoring through echocardiograms and managing cardiovascular risk factors are important.

- **Diarrhea:** Staying hydrated, eating a bland diet, and using anti-diarrheal medications can help manage diarrhea. Consulting a dietitian for specific dietary recommendations may also be beneficial.

6.5 General Strategies for Managing Side Effects

- **Pain Management:** Over-the-counter pain relievers, prescription medications, and complementary therapies like acupuncture and massage can help manage pain.
- **Emotional and Psychological Support:** Support groups, counseling, and therapy can provide emotional support. Mindfulness, meditation, and stress management techniques can also help cope with the psychological impact of treatment.

- **Nutrition:** A balanced diet rich in fruits, vegetables, lean proteins, and whole grains supports overall health and helps manage treatment side effects. Consulting a nutritionist can provide personalized dietary guidance.

Managing the side effects of breast cancer treatment is a multifaceted approach involving medications, lifestyle adjustments, and supportive therapies. Effective side effect management enhances quality of life and helps patients maintain strength and resilience throughout their treatment journey. Regular communication with healthcare providers ensures timely interventions and support tailored to individual needs.

CHAPTER 7

Survivorship and Follow-Up Care for Breast Cancer

Survivorship in breast cancer begins the moment treatment concludes, marking a new phase focused on recovery, monitoring, and maintaining health. Effective follow-up care is crucial for early detection of recurrence, managing long-term side effects, and addressing the emotional and psychological needs of survivors.

7.1 Regular Monitoring

1. Medical Check-Ups: Regular follow-up appointments are essential. Typically, survivors see their oncologist every three to six months for the first few years after treatment, then annually.

These visits often include a physical examination, discussion of symptoms, and updates on overall health.

2. Imaging Tests: Mammograms are recommended annually for both the treated and untreated breast. Additional imaging, such as MRIs or ultrasounds, may be required based on individual risk factors and previous cancer characteristics.

3. Blood Tests: Blood tests may be conducted to monitor overall health and check for markers indicating cancer recurrence. These tests can include complete blood counts, liver function tests, and tumor markers if necessary.

7.2 Managing Long-Term Side Effects

1. Lymphedema: Swelling due to lymph node removal or radiation can be managed through physical therapy, compression garments, and exercises to promote lymphatic drainage.

2. Bone Health: Treatments like hormone therapy can affect bone density. Survivors should ensure adequate calcium and vitamin D intake, engage in weight-bearing exercises, and undergo regular bone density scans.

3. Cardiovascular Health: Certain treatments can impact heart health. Regular cardiovascular screenings and adopting heart-healthy habits, such as a balanced diet and regular exercise, are essential.

7.3 Emotional and Psychological Support

1. Mental Health: Survivors often face anxiety, depression, and fear of recurrence. Counseling, support groups, and mental health professionals can provide necessary emotional support.

2. Quality of Life: Addressing issues like fatigue, cognitive changes (often called "chemo brain"), and changes in body image are important. Survivors should be encouraged to engage in activities that promote mental and physical well-being.

7.4 Lifestyle Adjustments

1. Healthy Diet: A diet rich in fruits, vegetables, whole grains, and lean proteins supports overall health. Limiting alcohol, avoiding tobacco, and maintaining a healthy weight are critical for reducing the risk of recurrence.

2. Physical Activity: Regular exercise helps manage weight, reduces fatigue, and improves overall health. Activities like walking, swimming, and yoga can be beneficial.

7.5 Preventive Measures

1. Screening for Other Cancers: Survivors should undergo regular screenings for other cancers as recommended, based on their treatment history and genetic predispositions.

2. Genetic Counseling: For those with a family history or genetic predispositions, genetic counseling and testing can provide information on risk and guide preventive measures for family members.

Survivorship and follow-up care for breast cancer involve comprehensive, ongoing management to detect recurrence early, mitigate long-term side effects, and address psychological and lifestyle factors. Regular monitoring, healthy lifestyle choices, and emotional support are pivotal in ensuring that survivors lead healthy, fulfilling lives post-treatment. Continuous communication with healthcare providers ensures that any new issues are promptly addressed, contributing to overall well-being and improved quality of life.

CHAPTER 8

Nutrition And Lifestyle

Maintaining a healthy diet and lifestyle is crucial for both the prevention and management of breast cancer. Proper nutrition and positive lifestyle choices can help reduce the risk of recurrence, improve treatment outcomes, and enhance overall well-being.

8.1 Nutrition

1. Balanced Diet: A diet rich in fruits, vegetables, whole grains, lean proteins, and healthy fats supports overall health. These foods provide essential vitamins, minerals, and antioxidants that can help combat cancer and boost the immune system.

2. Plant-Based Foods: Emphasizing plant-based foods, such as fruits, vegetables, legumes, and nuts, can provide phytonutrients and fiber that may have protective effects against cancer.

Cruciferous vegetables (like broccoli and Brussels sprouts) and berries are particularly beneficial due to their high antioxidant content.

3. Healthy Fats: Incorporating healthy fats, such as those found in olive oil, avocados, nuts, and fatty fish (like salmon), can reduce inflammation and support heart health. Omega-3 fatty acids, in particular, have been linked to lower cancer risk.

4. Limiting Processed Foods and Sugars: Reducing intake of processed foods, sugary beverages, and refined carbohydrates can help maintain a healthy weight and reduce cancer risk. These foods can lead to obesity and insulin resistance, which are linked to higher cancer risk.

5. Moderation in Alcohol: Alcohol consumption should be limited, as even moderate drinking can increase the risk of breast cancer. Women should aim for no more than one drink per day, if at all.

8.2 Lifestyle

1. Regular Physical Activity: Engaging in regular physical activity, such as brisk walking, swimming, or yoga, helps maintain a healthy weight, reduces fatigue, and improves mood. Aim for at least 150 minutes of moderate exercise or 75 minutes of vigorous exercise per week.

2. Healthy Weight: Maintaining a healthy weight is crucial, as obesity is a significant risk factor for breast cancer recurrence. Weight management through diet and exercise is essential.

3. Stress Reduction: Managing stress through activities like meditation, deep breathing exercises, and hobbies can improve mental health and overall well-being. Chronic stress can negatively impact the immune system and overall health.

4. Avoiding Tobacco: Tobacco use is linked to various cancers, including breast cancer. Quitting smoking improves overall health and reduces cancer risk.

Adopting a balanced diet and healthy lifestyle can significantly impact breast cancer outcomes. Regular physical activity, maintaining a healthy weight, managing stress, and avoiding harmful substances are key strategies for reducing risk and enhancing overall health. These lifestyle changes not only support cancer prevention but also contribute to a better quality of life for those living with and beyond breast cancer.

CHAPTER 9

Prevention and Risk Reduction

Breast cancer prevention and risk reduction involve a combination of lifestyle modifications, regular screening, and in some cases, medical interventions. While some risk factors like genetics and age cannot be controlled, there are several strategies that can significantly reduce the risk of developing breast cancer.

9.1 Lifestyle Modifications

1. Maintain a Healthy Weight: Obesity, especially after menopause, is a significant risk factor for breast cancer. Maintaining a healthy weight through a balanced diet and regular exercise can help reduce this risk. Aim for a body mass index (BMI) within the normal range.

2. Regular Physical Activity: Engaging in regular physical activity helps control weight,

reduces inflammation, and lowers estrogen levels, all of which can reduce breast cancer risk. The American Cancer Society recommends at least 150 minutes of moderate exercise or 75 minutes of vigorous exercise per week.

3. Healthy Diet: A diet rich in fruits, vegetables, whole grains, and lean proteins can support overall health and potentially reduce cancer risk. Foods high in antioxidants, such as berries and leafy greens, and healthy fats from sources like olive oil and fish, can be particularly beneficial.

4. Limit Alcohol Consumption: Alcohol intake is linked to an increased risk of breast cancer. Limiting alcohol consumption to no more than one drink per day for women can help reduce this risk.

5. Avoid Tobacco:Smoking is associated with an increased risk of many cancers, including breast cancer. Quitting smoking improves overall health and reduces cancer risk.

9.2 Medical Interventions

1. Regular Screening: Regular screening, such as mammograms, can detect breast cancer at an early stage when it is most treatable. Women should discuss with their healthcare providers the appropriate age and frequency for screening based on their risk factors.

2. Genetic Testing and Counseling: Women with a family history of breast cancer may benefit from genetic testing for BRCA1, BRCA2, and other gene mutations. Genetic counseling can help assess risk and guide decisions about preventive measures.

3. Chemoprevention: For women at high risk, medications like tamoxifen and raloxifene can reduce the risk of developing breast cancer. These drugs block or reduce estrogen's effects on breast tissue, which can lower the risk of hormone receptor-positive breast cancer.

4. Preventive Surgery: In very high-risk cases, such as those with BRCA1 or BRCA2 mutations, preventive (prophylactic) mastectomy or oophorectomy (removal of the ovaries) may be considered to significantly reduce the risk of developing breast and ovarian cancer.

9.3 Environmental Factors

1. Limit Radiation Exposure: Avoiding unnecessary medical imaging tests and taking protective measures when exposure is necessary can reduce the risk associated with ionizing radiation.

2. Reduce Exposure to Environmental Toxins: Limiting exposure to certain chemicals found in some plastics, cosmetics, and household products may help lower cancer risk. Choosing products free of known carcinogens can be beneficial.

Breast cancer prevention and risk reduction involve a multifaceted approach, including lifestyle modifications, regular screening, and in some cases, medical interventions. By maintaining a healthy weight, staying physically active, eating a balanced diet, limiting alcohol, avoiding tobacco, and considering genetic testing and preventive medications, individuals can significantly reduce their risk of developing breast cancer. Regular communication with healthcare providers ensures personalized and effective strategies for prevention.

CHAPTER 10

Support And Resources

Navigating a breast cancer diagnosis and treatment can be overwhelming. Having a strong support system and access to comprehensive resources is crucial for emotional well-being and practical assistance. Here's an overview of various support systems and resources available for breast cancer patients and their families:

10.1 Emotional and Psychological Support

- **Family and Friends:** The support of loved ones is invaluable. They can provide emotional comfort, practical help, and companionship. Encouraging open communication about feelings and needs helps build a strong support network.

- **Support Groups:** Joining a support group allows patients to connect with others going through similar experiences. These groups provide a safe space to share fears, challenges, and successes. They can be found through hospitals, community centers, or online platforms.

- **Counseling and Therapy**: Professional counselors or therapists specializing in oncology can help patients and their families cope with the emotional toll of cancer. Therapy can address anxiety, depression, and stress management, offering strategies for emotional resilience.

10.2 Practical and Financial Support

- **Patient Navigators:** Patient navigators help guide individuals through the healthcare system, coordinating appointments, and providing information on treatment options and resources. They can be found in many cancer treatment centers and hospitals.

- **Financial Assistance Programs:** The cost of cancer treatment can be substantial. Organizations like the American Cancer Society, Susan G. Komen, and CancerCare offer financial assistance for medical expenses, transportation, and daily living costs. Patients should also consult with hospital social workers to explore available resources.

- **Legal Resources:** Legal issues related to employment, insurance, and disability can arise. Organizations such as the Cancer Legal Resource Center provide free legal information and support to navigate these challenges.

10.3 Educational Resources

- **Educational Workshops and Seminars:** Many cancer centers and organizations offer workshops on topics such as treatment options, nutrition, and coping strategies. These programs empower patients with knowledge to make informed decisions.

- **Reliable Online Resources:** Websites like the American Cancer Society, Breastcancer.org, and the National Cancer Institute offer comprehensive information on breast cancer, including treatment options, side effects, and survivorship.

10.4 Complementary Therapies

- **Integrative Medicine:** Integrative medicine combines conventional treatments with complementary therapies such as acupuncture, massage, and meditation. These therapies can help manage side effects, reduce stress, and improve overall well-being.

- **Nutrition and Exercise Programs:** Registered dietitians and fitness experts can provide tailored advice to help manage treatment side effects and improve strength and energy levels. Many cancer centers offer specialized nutrition and exercise programs for their patients.

10.5 Community Resources

- **Local Community Services:** Community organizations often provide practical support, such as transportation to treatment, meal delivery, and home care services. These services can greatly ease the burden on patients and their families.

- **Religious and Spiritual Support:** For those who find comfort in faith, spiritual care providers can offer emotional and spiritual support. Many hospitals have chaplains or can connect patients with local religious organizations.

A robust support system and access to diverse resources are essential for managing breast cancer's physical, emotional, and practical challenges. Leveraging family, friends, professional counselors, patient navigators, financial aid, educational resources, and complementary therapies can significantly enhance the quality of life for breast cancer patients. Regular communication with healthcare providers ensures that patients receive comprehensive care tailored to their unique needs.

CONCLUSION

Breast cancer remains a significant health challenge, affecting millions worldwide. However, advancements in detection, treatment, and support have greatly improved outcomes and survivorship. Early detection through regular screenings and awareness of risk factors is critical for effective treatment. Comprehensive treatment plans, including surgery, radiation, chemotherapy, and targeted therapies, offer personalized approaches to combat the disease.

Equally important is the support system surrounding patients. Emotional, practical, and financial support from family, friends, healthcare professionals, and community organizations plays a crucial role in the journey to recovery. Integrative therapies, nutrition, and exercise further enhance quality of life and overall well-being.

Awareness and education are vital in the fight against breast cancer. By staying informed about prevention strategies, risk factors, and available resources, individuals can take proactive steps to reduce their risk and seek timely medical advice.

Ultimately, a holistic approach that combines medical treatment with emotional and practical support can empower individuals to navigate breast cancer with strength and resilience. Continued research and community support will drive further progress, offering hope and improved outcomes for all affected by this disease.